Powerful Mamas®

DIY Placenta Encapsulation Guide + Bonus Items

A How-To Guide for Raw, TCM and Basic Heated Methods of Preparation

Jacquelyn Duke, CPES(IPPA)

Copyright © 2014 Intrinsic Birthing LLC

All rights reserved.

ISBN: 1515070247
ISBN-13: 978-1515070245

DEDICATION

To my greatest loves, Willow & Maya…and the amazing daddy who made them possible!

CONTENTS

	Acknowledgments	i
1	Part 1: Important Considerations Prior to DIY Placenta Encapsulation	1
2	Part 2: Proper Handling of the Placenta Immediately After Birth	2
3	Part 3: Safety Recommendations for During the Encapsulation Process	4
4	Part 4: Supplies Needed for Encapsulation	6
5	Part 5: Beginning Phase 1 of the Encapsulation Process - Preparing the Placenta for Dehydration, Creating Tree of Life Prints, Designing an Umbilical Cord Keepsake, Making a Placenta Recovery Broth, and Prepping the Placenta Tincture	8
6	Part 6: Beginning Phase 2 of the Encapsulation Process – Grinding and Encapsulating the Placenta	29
7	Powerful Mamas Healing Placenta Salve Recipe	31
8	Powerful Mamas Placenta Smoothie Recipe	32
9	About the Author	33
10	Disclaimer	34

ACKNOWLEDGMENTS

As a labor and postpartum doula, childbirth educator and placenta encapsulationist, I have had the incredible honor of bearing witness to the strength of the human body during pregnancy, birth and beyond. I would like to thank all of my clients, both past and present, that have allowed me to learn alongside them on their journeys into parenthood. Perhaps one of the greatest lessons I have embraced over the years is this: There is often more than one way to reach our destination. If we can be open to new possibilities, adventures, and challenges, we often can achieve things we never thought possible before…

I admire your willingness to try new things! Please join me as I share with you how YOU can harness the power of the placenta, right from the comfort of your own home!

1
PART 1: IMPORTANT CONSIDERATIONS PRIOR TO DIY PLACENTA ENCAPSULATION

When handling any blood products, it is highly suggested the handler take OSHA Certified blood borne pathogens training. While it is true the mother cannot pass a blood borne disease to herself during preparation, it is important proper cleaning procedures are followed for the sake of others that may come into contact with the space in which the placenta is prepared. It is especially important that anyone handling the placenta other than the mother be aware of proper safety procedures to avoid the spread of disease. Biologix offers an excellent and inexpensive online training found here:http://blxtraining.com/placenta-encapsulation-specialists/ . As a Powerful Mamas customer you may enter coupon code "placenta" to receive $5 off the training price!

      Remember that the placenta should be handled just as carefully as any other meat one plans to consume. The preparer should abide by proper food safety recommendations at all times for storage and preparation. If the preparer is uncertain about proper food handling procedures it is highly recommended they take a training course on food safety prior to performing placenta encapsulation. Each state offers inexpensive online training, such as the Food Handler Training found from Servsafe® at http://www.servsafe.com/foodhandler/.

2
PART 2: PROPER HANDLING OF THE PLACENTA IMMEDIATELY AFTER BIRTH

Make sure your healthcare provider understands that the mother wants to keep her placenta for consumption. It may be helpful to include this on a birth plan and to discuss it with the provider prior to the birth. Ask about any hospital policies that might exist regarding release of the placenta. Offer to sign any required release forms prior to the birth, if possible.

Cool the placenta IMMEDIATELY after the birth by either freezing it for preparation at one's convenience, or by placing it in a refrigerator at 30-40 degrees Fahrenheit for no more than 3-5 days prior to preparation. Prepare the placenta immediately once taken out of the refrigerator. If frozen, thaw the placenta in the refrigerator, (NOT on the counter!), then prepare the placenta shortly after thawing is complete. Do not refreeze the thawed placenta. It is recommended that the placenta is prepared fresh to retain the most hormonal benefits. If the mother must freeze the placenta prepare it as soon as possible, but no later than 6 months postpartum.

Always verify with the mother's health care provider the safety of the placenta for consumption. Certain conditions can make the placenta unsafe to consume, such as a bacterial infection before or during the birth, or improper storage or handling of the placenta after the birth. (Please note that excessive meconium CAN be a contraindication for encapsulation, though many mothers have chosen to encapsulate in the presence of meconium after a thorough rinse with cold water and a vinegar bath, using only the basic heated method. Exercise good judgment in the case of meconium, depending on the severity and the health care provider's recommendations.)

Verify the placenta did not come into contact with any chemicals, such as bleach or formaldehyde, at any time - particularly if the placenta left the mother's presence and/or went to the pathology department of the hospital. If the placenta needs to be tested the mother can request that only a small piece be taken rather than the entire placenta. Keeping the placenta in the mother's presence at all times is the best way to insure it has been handled properly. The mother may want to bring a cooler to the birth if there is not reliable access to a secure refrigerator; but be aware that the ice in the cooler must be changed ***every 4 hours,*** and the placenta still must be moved to a refrigerator within 12 hours to avoid spoilage.

If it is determined that the placenta is unsafe to consume, keep in mind one can still prepare beautiful placenta prints and an umbilical cord keepsake as a lasting memory of this incredible, life-giving organ. <u>Powerful Mamas' DIY Placenta Encapsulation Kit provides all of the materials to do these keepsakes, in addition to the materials needed for encapsulation!</u>

Most hospitals or birthing centers will provide the mother with a red biohazard plastic bag or container to take the placenta home. Check that the hospital has labeled the placenta with the correct name, date of birth, and address prior to transport.

3
PART 3: SAFETY RECOMMENDATIONS FOR DURING THE ENCAPSULATION PROCESS

Clean all work surfaces thoroughly prior to the encapsulation, as well as in between phases while the placenta is dehydrating, and after the entire process is done. Begin by using antibacterial soap, followed by a recognized kitchen grade cleaning agent, such as Lysol. It is recommended one follow cleaning procedures with a 9 parts water to 1 part household bleach solution applied for at least 20 minutes before and after all phases of the encapsulation process, in order to reduce the risk of blood borne pathogens. Be sure to use an UNOPENED bottle of bleach. Rinse and wash any food surfaces and utensils free of bleach prior to use. Learn more about decontamination procedures for blood here: http://www.cdc.gov/healthywater/swimming/pools/cleaning-body-fluid-spills.html.

    Always change into a clean pair of gloves AND use a clean prep space and clean knife when transitioning from handling a raw placenta to a steamed placenta. Use a fresh absorbent pad as well. Do not cross contaminate raw meat prep surfaces with steamed meat surfaces! Wash hands and change into clean gloves if one use's the restroom, sneezes, wipes the nose, or otherwise contaminates one's hands. Consider wearing a handkerchief over the mouth and nose or a face mask during the grinding process to avoid inhalation of the placenta, especially if using an electric grinder instead of the mortar and pestle provided in ***Powerful Mamas' DIY Placenta Preparation Kit***. Exercise extreme caution when handling hot items and sharp knives throughout the encapsulation process! Always keep the knife facing away from the body at all times.

4
PART 4: SUPPLIES NEEDED FOR ENCAPSULATION

You will need the following items to complete the encapsulation process, and to make the bonus items of a cord keepsake, tree of life placenta prints, placenta recovery broth, and a placenta tincture. *All of these supplies are included in Powerful Mamas DIY Placenta Encapsulation Kit.* If you have only purchased this manual and have decided you'd like to go ahead and order the full kit, please use coupon code "SAVE10" for ten percent off your kit at www.PowerfulMamas.com!

Powerful Mamas DIY Placenta Encapsulation Supply List:

- 1 Five to 8 Qt. Stockpot with Lid (For Rinsing and Steaming Placenta)
- 1 Tin Cake Pan (To be Punctured and Used in Bottom of Pot UPSIDE DOWN to create a platform for Steaming the Placenta)
- 1 Small Plastic Bowl (For Placing Grinded Placenta Powder)
- 4 Pairs Nitrile Gloves (Wear Fresh Gloves at Each Stage of Encapsulation)
- 1 Blue Glass 4 Ounce Bottle (For Placenta Tincture)
- 4 ounces of 100 Proof Alcohol for Placenta Tincture (*Not Included in Powerful Mamas DIY Placenta Encapsulation Kit Due to Shipping Restrictions)

DIY Placenta Encapsulation Guide

- 1 Organza Keepsake Bag (For Storing Umbilical Cord Keepsake)
- 1 Quart Freezer Bag (For Storing Frozen Placenta Recovery Broth Frozen Cubes)
- 1 Face Mask (To Wear During Grinding & Encapsulation, If Desired)
- 1 Blue Plastic Storage Jar for Finished Placenta Capsules
- 150-250 Empty Size 0 Vegetable Capsules
- 1 Food Safe Desiccant Packet (To Be Placed In Finished Placenta Capsules Jar to Reduce Humidity)
- 1 Mortar & Pestle (For Grinding the Placenta into Powder – You May Choose to Use an Electric Grinder Instead)
- 3 Chuck Pads (To Be Used Under Cutting Boards and During Grinding Process for Easy Cleanup)
- 6 Sheets of Paper Towels (To Prep the Placenta for Watercolor Prints)
- 1 Dinner Fork (Used to Puncture Tin Steaming Pan, to Remove the Placenta from the Steaming Pot, & for Slicing the Placenta)
- 1 Colander for Rinsing the Raw Placenta
- 1 Chef Knife
- 1 Meat Thermometer (To Check Internal Temperature of the Steamed Placenta)
- 1 Encapsulation Machine (Or You May Choose to Encapsulate By Hand)
- 2 Cutting Boards (Use One for the Raw Placenta and One for the Steamed Placenta)
- 2 Sheets of Aluminum Foil, Each 20" Long (For Wrapping/Lining Oven Racks, OR 2 Disposable, Tin Cookie Sheets, OR You May Choose to Use Your Own Food Dehydrator)
- 2 Sheets of Parchment Paper, Each 12"x16" (Placed on Top of Foil, Cookie Sheets, or Food Dehydrator Trays while Dehydrating the Placenta for Easy Clean Up)
- 4 Water Color Papers (For Making Placenta Prints)
- 1 Ice Cube Tray (For Freezing Placenta Recovery Broth)

5
PART 5: BEGINNING PHASE 1 OF THE ENCAPSULATION PROCESS!

(Allow 1-2 hours to prepare the placenta and bonus items for dehydration. Allow an additional 3-4 hours for monitoring the oven.)

Please note that these instructions are directed towards the mother, with the assumption that she is the one preparing her own placenta.

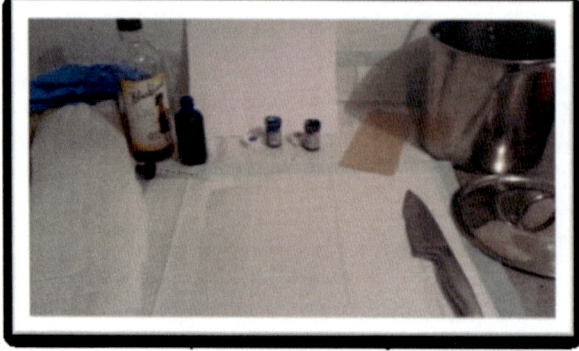

Step 1: After Cleaning & Sanitizing Your Work Surface, Organize your Materials & Prep Space.

Place the cutting board on top of the chuck pad so it can catch spills. Place all materials within reach. Make sure you are near a water source, a stove top, and an oven.

Step 2: Open the Placenta Container.

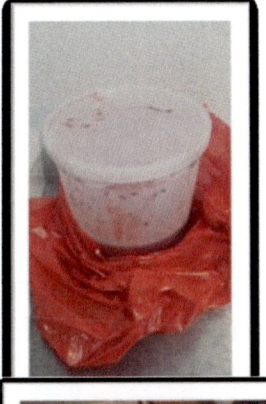

Your placenta should have been given to you in a labeled container with a red biohazard bag or container holding it.

Step 3: Become Familiar with the Placenta

- The Fetal Side:

The smooth side of the placenta is known as the fetal side. It is the side that faced and connected to your baby via the umbilical cord.

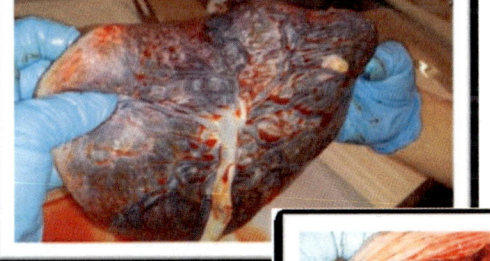

- The Maternal Side:

The bumpy, meaty side of the placenta is known as the maternal side. It connected to your uterus.

Become Familiar with the Placenta - The Amniotic Sac.

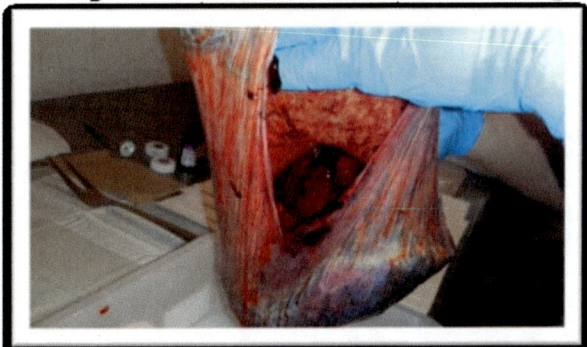

The amniotic sac may or may not have begun to separate from your placenta. The sac is what surrounded your baby and held your amniotic fluid.

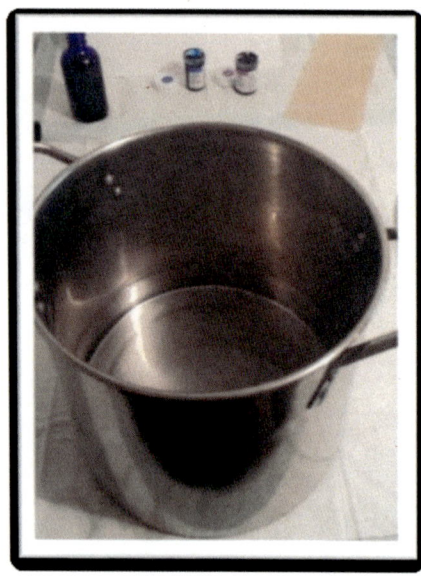

Step 4: Gently Rinse the Placenta & Umbilical Cord.

You may use the stock pot to rinse the placenta under running water, or you may use a colander to rinse the placenta under running water. Remove any large blood clots. Discard all blood products in the biohazard bag provided by your health practitioner.

*If the baby passed meconium prior to birth and your provider has approved the placenta for encapsulation, be sure to rinse off all fecal matter. Remove and discard the amniotic sac. If there is still green or brown staining, use 1 Tbsp. Apple cider vinegar to remove staining on the placenta and the umbilical cord. Rinse with water. Raw encapsulation is NOT recommended if there was meconium found on the placenta!

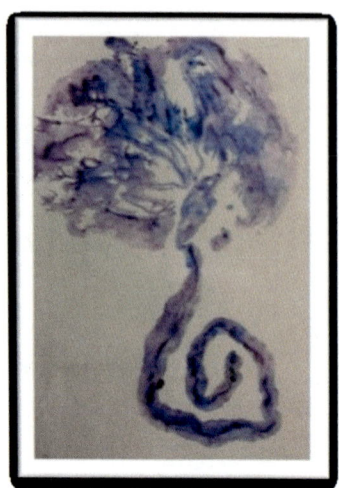

Step 5: Decide if you would like to make Placenta Prints. If not, skip to Step 18.

*Placenta prints can be done even if the placenta cannot be consumed. They are a wonderful option with or without encapsulation!

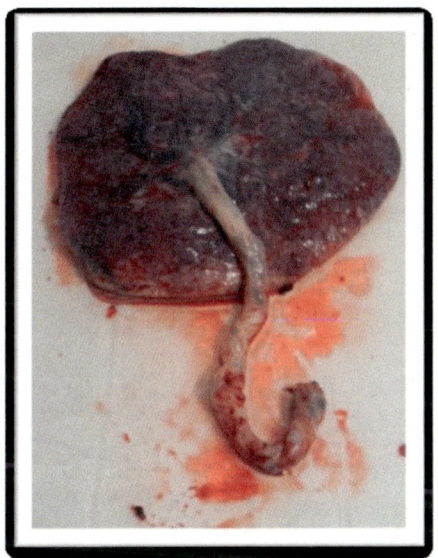

Step 6: Place the Placenta Maternal Side Down on the Disposable Cutting Board

For Placenta Prints, you can either remove the amniotic sac, or tuck it underneath the maternal side of the placenta while doing the prints. Clean up any blood splatters on the cutting board using a paper towel so that they do not interfere with your print.

Step 7: Prepare the Placenta for Printing.

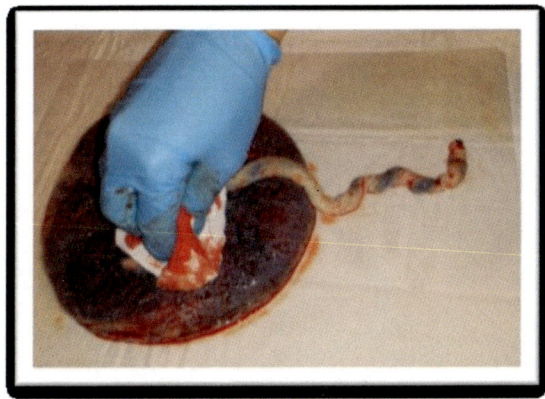

Blot the fetal (smooth) side of the placenta to remove excess water, blood and any small clots remaining. To make natural prints, add some fresh blood by dipping your gloved fingertips into the container the placenta came in, then gently spread the blood like paint over the placenta and cord. Have fun arranging the umbilical cord in various patterns! If there is enough cord, you could try making a heart, a swirl, or just make the cord look like the trunk of a tree. After all, the placenta is often referred to as the tree of life!

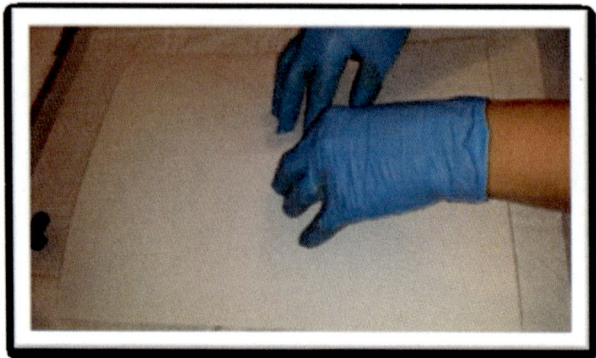

Step 8: Place the Watercolor Paper on Top of the Placenta.

Tap GENTLY with dry fingertips, being sure to press along the umbilical cord and all the way out to the edges of the placenta.

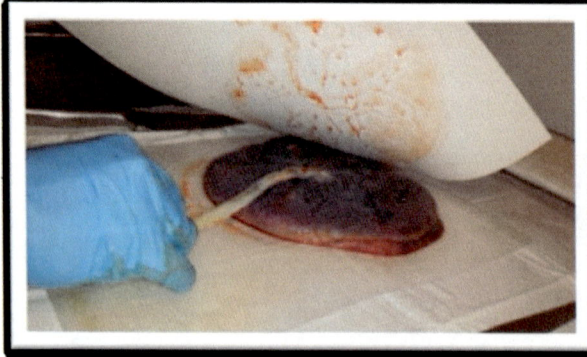

Step 9: Starting at the Bottom Corner, Gently Peel Back the Water Color Paper.

The umbilical cord tends to stick, so hold the end firmly while lifting the paper with your other hand. Try not to smear the print! Lift carefully, pulling the paper away slowly from the placenta. Set the prints aside to dry.

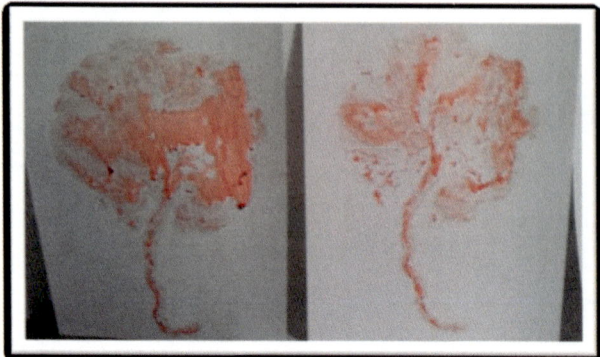

Step 10: Repeat the Process for a Sharper Image.

The first print is generally thicker. The second print often comes out better. If you are still getting a smeared look, try blotting away more fluid prior to printing.

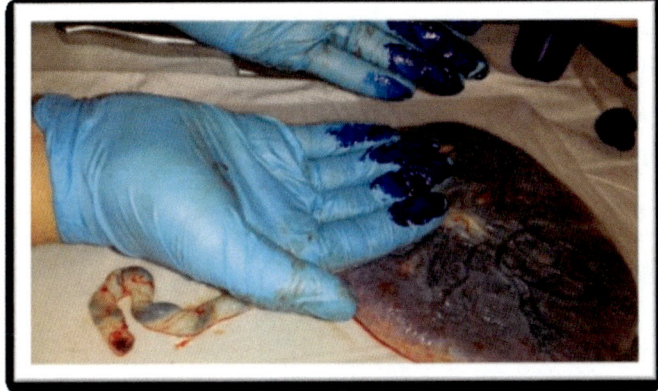

Step 11: OPTIONAL - Making Colored Prints with Natural or Commercial Food Coloring.

You may use natural, food safe items such as turmeric, spirulina, or beet powder mixed with a little water to make a paste, or you may also use any commercial food coloring to make colored prints. (Powerful Mamas prefers Wilton cake frosting food dyes for placenta prints!)

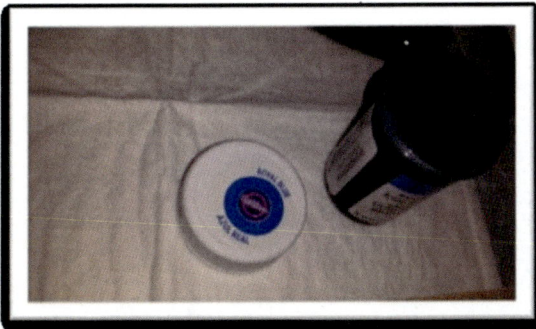

Step 12: Apply a Dime Size Amount of Food Coloring to Your Fingertips.

*Make sure the mother has no allergies to the food colorings prior to applying them directly to the placenta if she plans to consume it! Alternatively, you may place a piece of plastic wrap over the placenta to act as a barrier from the food coloring, but the image might not be as sharp.

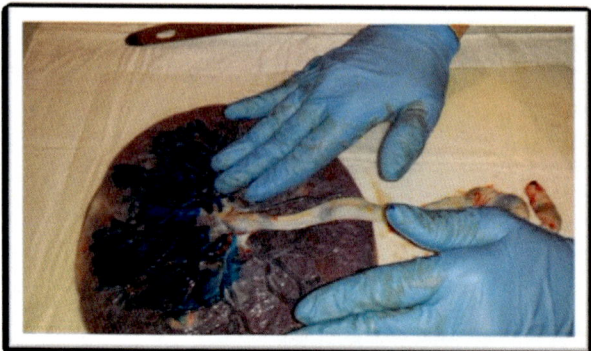

Step 13: Spread the Food Coloring Over the Surface of the Placenta. Make Sure to Cover the Main Veins of the Placenta.

Don't forget to dab some color on the umbilical cord!

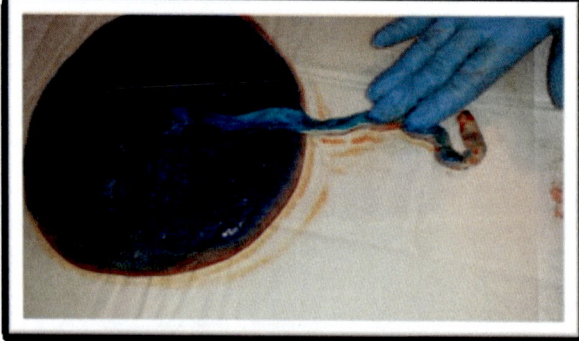

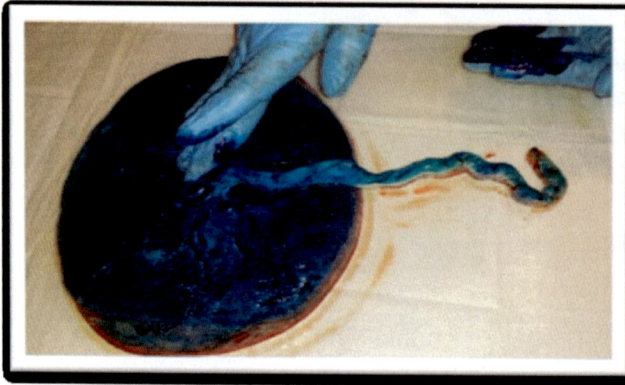

Step 14: For a Tie-Dye Effect, Add the Second Color to Your Fingertips.

Start at the base of the umbilical cord. Spread the food coloring outward, just along the main veins of the placenta. Don't forget to dab a little of the second color at various points on the cord!

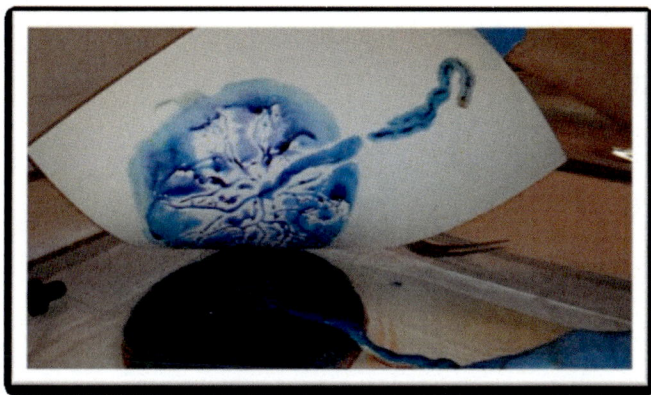

Step 15: Peel the Paper Back Slowly and Carefully.

Set the prints aside to dry in a safe location.

Step 16: Repeat the Process for a Second and Even Third Print.

Each print will become crisper as more color is removed from the placenta.

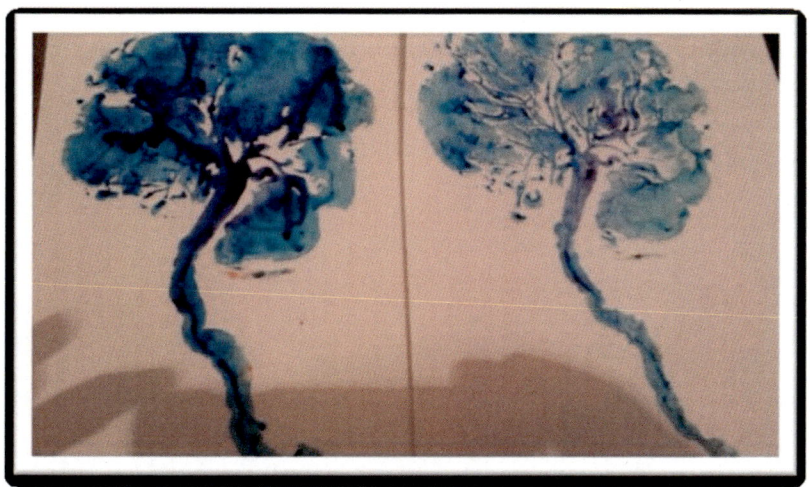

Step 17: Enjoy Your Masterpieces!

Placenta prints look beautiful on the wall of the nursery, as a conversation piece, or as a beautiful keepsake in the baby book!!!

Step 18: Remove the Umbilical Cord.

Holding the end of the cord firmly, place your knife at the base of the umbilical cord and cut away from your body. Be prepared for some blood to leak at the point of separation.

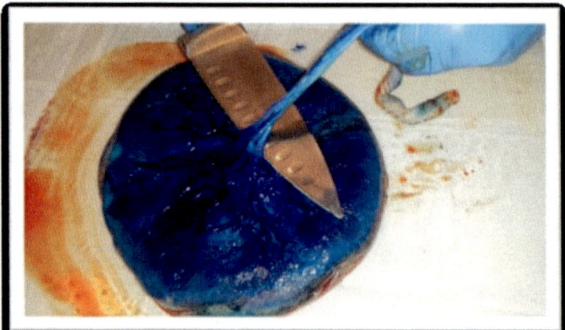

*Either discard the cord, encapsulate the cord after heating it with the placenta, or complete Steps 19-21 for making an umbilical cord keepsake

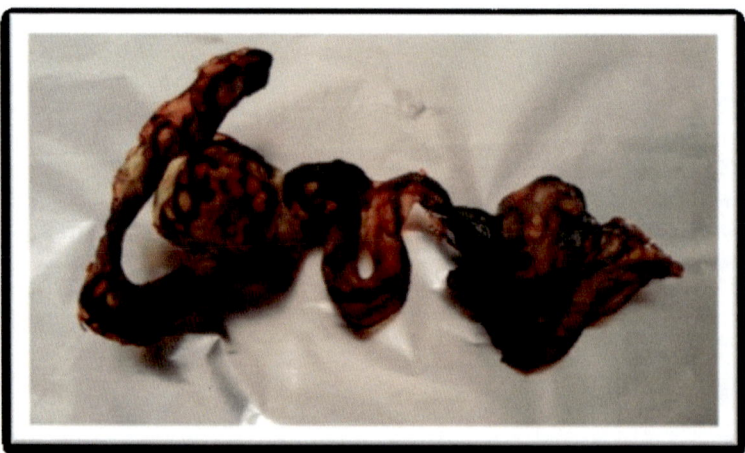

Step 19: Twist the Cord into a Desirable Shape on a Small Piece of Parchment Paper.

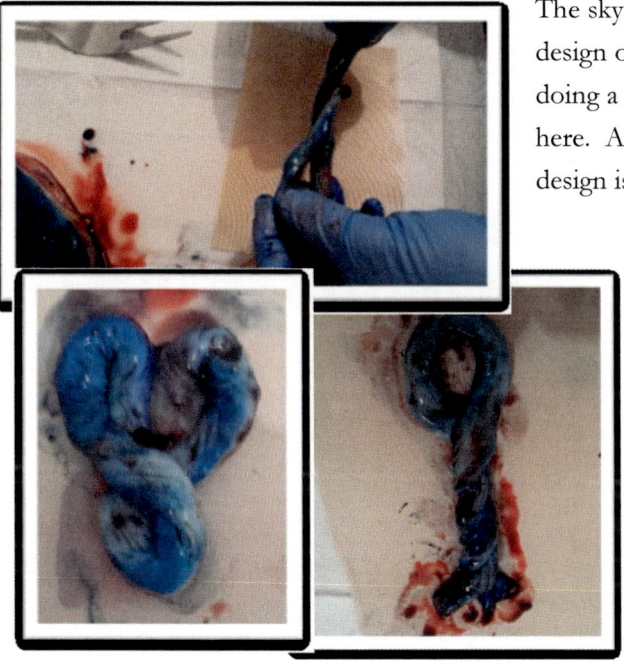

The sky is the limit for design options!!! Try doing a key, as shown here. Another popular design is a heart shape.

If you have a very short piece of cord, you might be best off doing a simple spiral or circle.

Step 20: Carefully Lift the Parchment Paper, Moving Your Keepsake Onto Either a Foil Wrapped Oven Rack, a Cookie Sheet, or a Dehydrator.

If continuing on with encapsulating your placenta, you may dehydrate the cord on the same paper, as pictured. Be sure to leave space all the

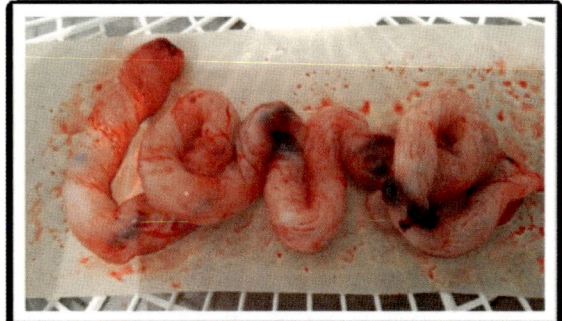

way around the cord, with no placenta touching the cord!

Follow dehydration instructions below for encapsulation. The cord should be crisp all the way through. <u>It should not bend, which indicates moisture</u>. Be careful when testing firmness not to break your keepsake!

Step 21: If Desired, Store Cord Keepsake in an Organza Keepsake Bag.

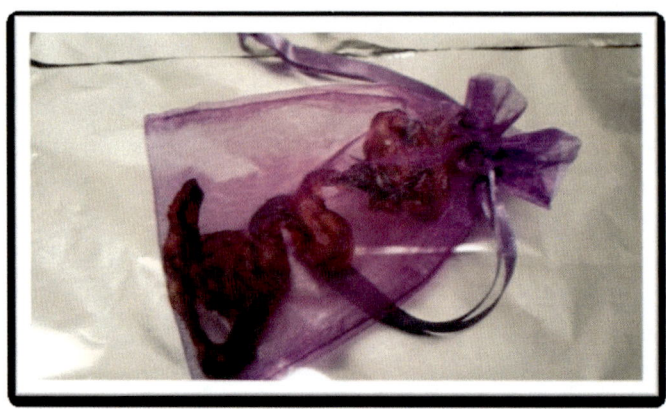

Step 22: Decide if You Will Be Making a Placenta Tincture. If so, complete Steps 23-27 at this point.

*You will need 4 ounces of 100 proof alcohol to complete the placenta tincture. Many choose apple brandy or rum, but any alcohol over 100 proof will do.

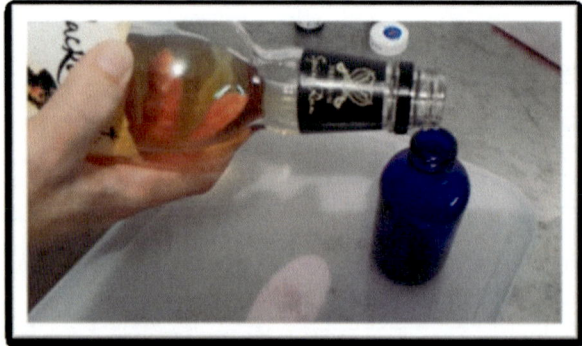

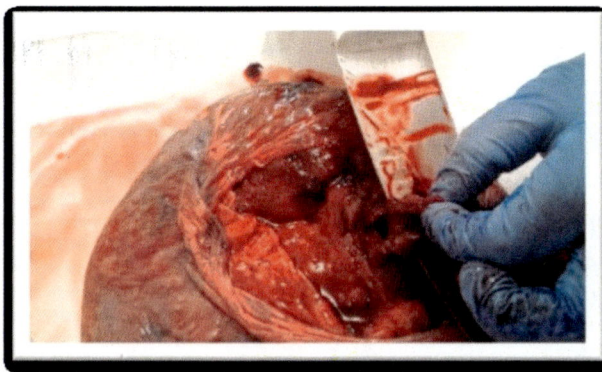

Step 23: Place the Placenta Maternal Side UP on the Disposable Cutting Board.

Step 24: Prepare the Placenta Tincture Bottle.

Fill the placenta tincture bottle with 100 proof liquor. (The high proof of the liquor will break down the raw placenta.)

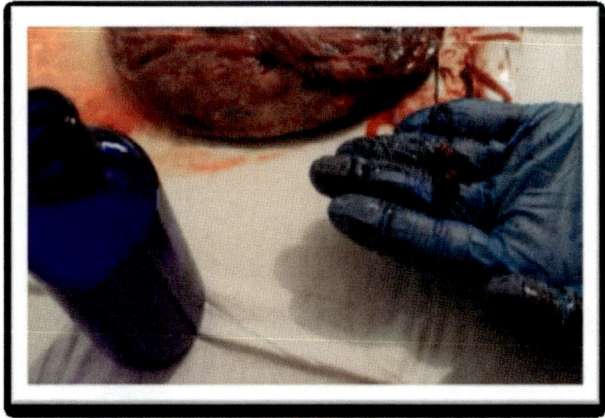

Step 25: Cutting Away from Your Body, Remove a Thumbnail-Sized Portion of Raw Placenta from the Placenta's Maternal Side.

Dice it small enough to fit into the top of the tincture bottle.

Step 26: Place this Small Portion into the Placenta Tincture Bottle.

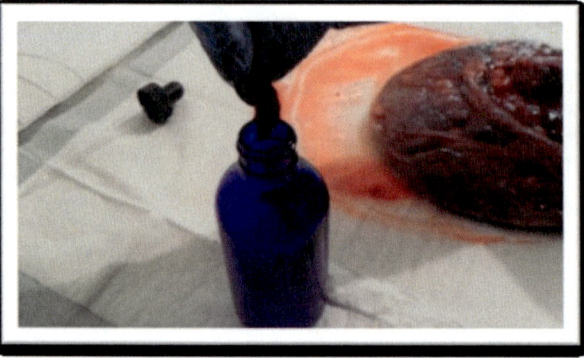

Place the dropper into the bottle and firmly tighten the lid.

Step 27: Place the Bottle in a Bright Window for 12 Hours. Then Move to a Cool, Dark Location.

It is suggested you wait at least 6 weeks before using the placenta tincture. You may strain the tincture prior to first use with a coffee filter, if desired, but it's not required. If prepared and stored properly, your tincture is shelf-stable indefinitely.

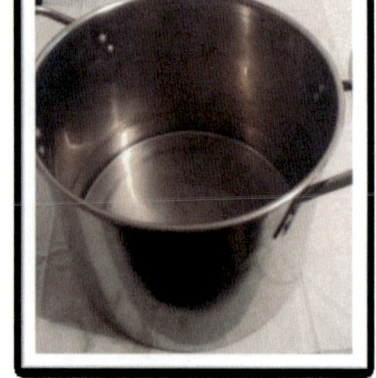

Step 28: Make Holes in the Foil Tin. Bend It to Fit in the Bottom of the Stock Pot. Fill the Stock Pot with Water Just Below the Top of the Foil Tin.

If using the basic-heated method, the placenta will rest on top of the foil pan as it steams.

*At this point some people choose to add herbs prescribed or recommended to them from a doctor of Chinese medicine to the water, so as to infuse the placenta and to include in the placenta recovery broth (described below)... <u>Herbs are not required in order to reap the benefits of placenta consumption, and should only be used under the direction of an experienced professional, such as a TCM doctor.</u>

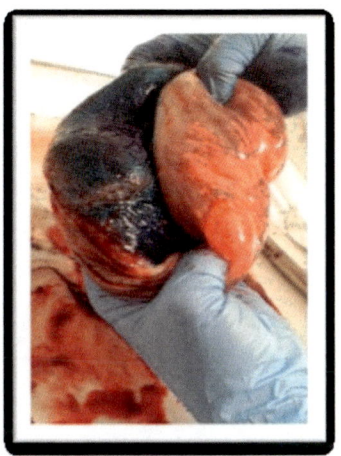

Step 29: Wrap the Placenta Inside the Amniotic Sac, if Possible.* IF DOING RAW ENCAPSULATION, SKIP TO STEP 37. (Powerful Mamas recommends using the basic heated method of preparation if meconium was present at birth, or if the placenta is older than 24 hours. Being GBS+ does not affect the method of encapsulation as long as you dehydrate at a minimum temperature of 160 degrees Fahrenheit, as recommended here)

Step 30: Begin Heating the Placenta.

Place the placenta gently on top of the foil tin in the stock pot. Put the lid on the stock pot and place it on the stove top on medium to medium high

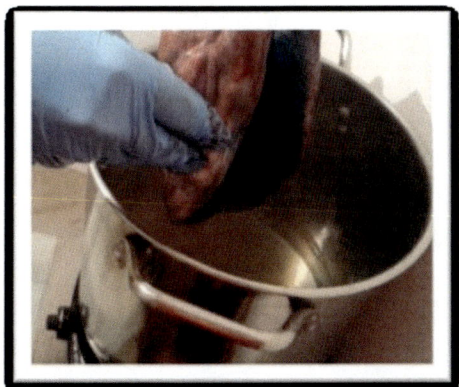

heat. Gently heat the placenta until it reaches an internal temperature of 160 degrees Fahrenheit. Check internal temperature using the meat thermometer. As the placenta heats, it will begin to curl. This is normal. Poke the placenta halfway through heating to release excess juices.

Step 31: When the Desired Temperature Has Been Reached, Remove the Placenta Using a Fork. It should be a medium-pink color in the middle – not raw, but not fully browned either. Place It to Cool On a New Cutting Board. Change Into New Gloves. *Exercise Caution! The placenta, pot and juices will be very hot!!! Allow everything to cool before handling.*

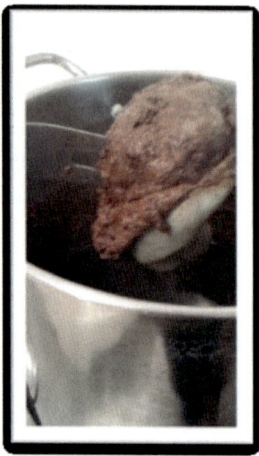

*After the pot has cooled enough to safely handle, place cooking water/placenta juices into the refrigerator. Refer to Steps 32-35 for directions on preparing a Placenta Recovery Broth for the mother.

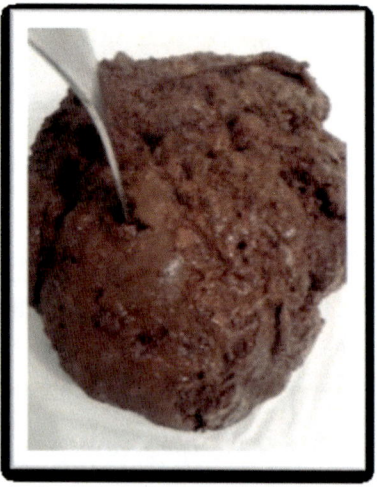

Step 32: Preparing a Placenta Recovery Broth.

Placenta recovery broths should be frozen in individual portions that can be easily thawed. An ice cube tray works well!

*As mentioned above, you may choose to infuse the Placenta Recovery Broth with herbs provided by a Doctor of Chinese Medicine. Just place the herbs in the water while heating the placenta. Alternatively, the herbs can be added to each individual serving of placenta recovery broth at the time of consumption. It is extremely important that you follow your TCM provider's recommendations for preparing any herbs added to your placenta recovery broth! It is NOT recommended that you add any herbs directly to your powdered placenta. If you have an adverse reaction to the herbs and they've been added to your capsules it could make your capsules unusable!

Step 33: Pour Cooled Placenta Recovery Broth (Washed Colandar Optional) into Individual Freezer Safe Containers, Such as Ice Cube Trays.

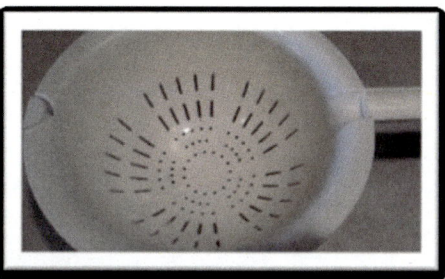

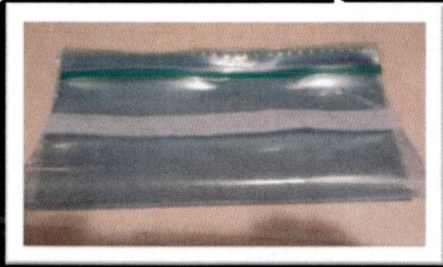

Step 34: Once Frozen, Move Placenta Broth Cubes Into a Freezer Safe Plastic Bag.

Label the bag with the mother's name, description of product, and the date the broth was made.

Step 35: Thaw and Consume Individual Servings of Placenta Recovery Broth as Desired.

A suggested daily intake of placenta recovery broth is 1 frozen cube mixed with 1 cup of warm water 1-2 times daily, the first ten days postpartum or until gone. Some women prefer to mix the broth with juice or add honey.
If infusing the broth with herbs, be sure to follow the dosage guidelines of your herbalist or TCM professional!

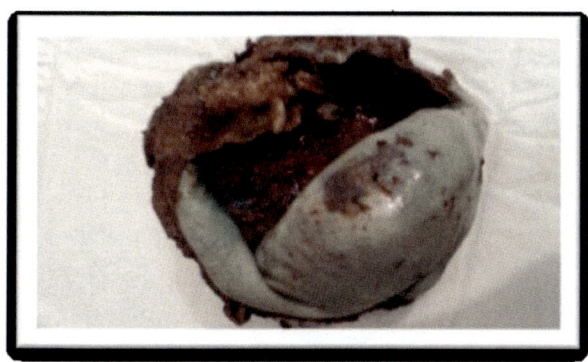

Step 36: Remove Any Excess Amniotic Sac from the Cooled Placenta, Cutting in a Circular Motion along the Outer Edge of the Placenta.

Place the amniotic sac on parchment paper for dehydration.

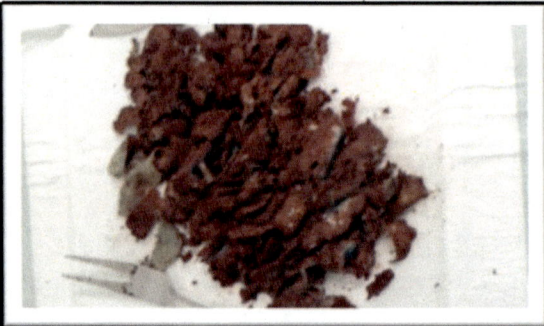

Step 37: Using a Fork and Knife, Slice the Placenta into Uniform, 1/8 Inch Thick Strips, No More Than 3 Inches Long.

Step 38: Prepare Oven Grill Racks.

Place foil over your oven grill racks, firmly squeezing around each end, or use cookie sheets. Place parchment paper on top of foil or cookie sheets to prevent sticking.

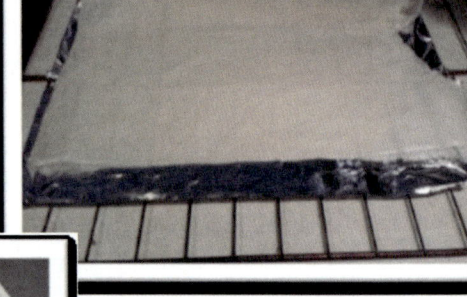

Optional: You may choose to use a food dehydrator instead of your oven. Cut to fit and place parchment paper on top of your dehydrator trays for easy clean up!

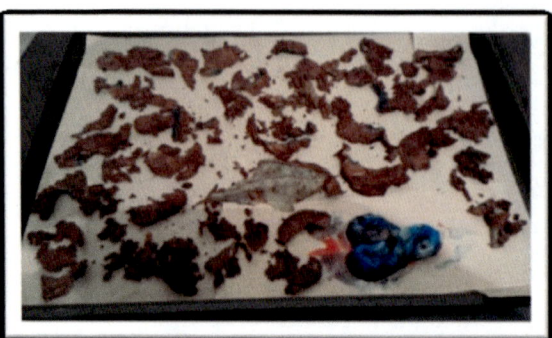

Step 39: Place Strips of Placenta on Parchment Paper, <u>Leaving Space between Each Strip for Adequate Air Circulation</u>.

Don't forget to place

the amniotic sac and the umbilical cord keepsake on the parchment paper! The amniotic sac and/or umbilical cord can be ground along with the placenta and placed in the placenta capsules if you prefer to encapsulate them along with the placenta.

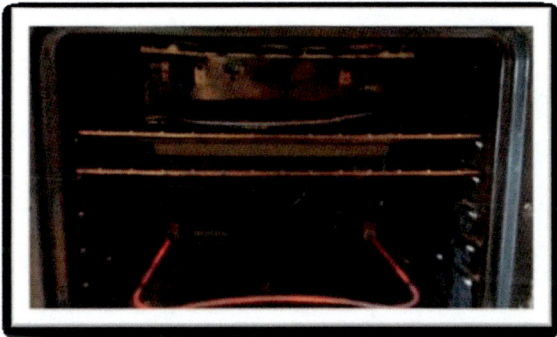

Step 40: Place Oven Racks at Top of Oven

Step 41: Heat Oven to 160-180 Degrees Fahrenheit. *(If using a food dehydrator, make sure you can set the dehydrator to 160 degrees Fahrenheit.)*

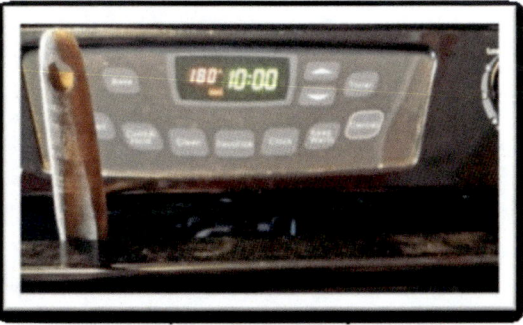

For food safety it is critical that you maintain a temperature of at least 160 degrees Fahrenheit for at least 2 hours to kill bacteria that could be present. Powerful Mamas keeps the temperature at 160 degrees for the entire length of encapsulation.

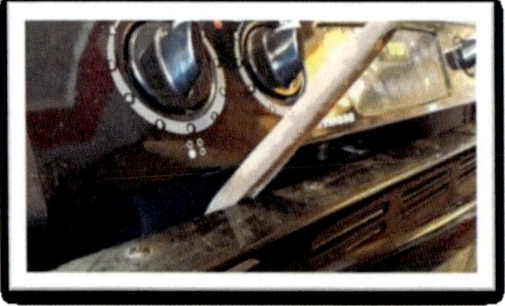

EXERCISE EXTREME CAUTION IF YOU CHOOSE TO PROP THE OVEN DOOR OPEN! Make sure no children or pets have access!!!

Depending on your oven, you may need to place a heat resistant spoon in the oven door to maintain the recommended temperature.

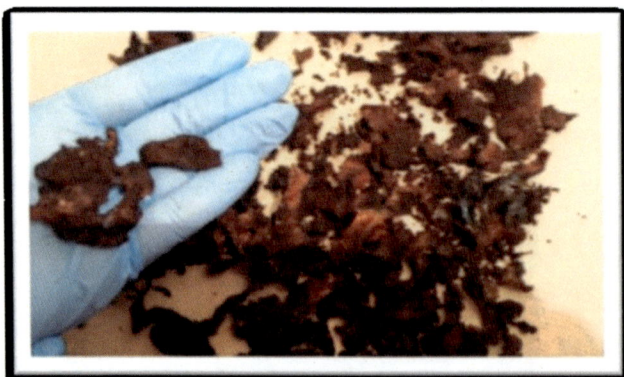

Step 42: Watch the Placenta CLOSELY. Remove It from the Oven When It Has Reached the Desired Consistency. Be Careful Not to Burn the Placenta in the Oven – You Are Attempting to Dry It, Not Bake It!!!

The placenta jerky should be crisp all the way through. It should not bend, and there should be no pink - both indicate moisture, which can lead to bacterial growth and/or mold! <u>It is critical for preservation purposes that each piece of jerky snaps.</u> *Ovens generally take 2-4 hours to fully dehydrate the placenta, but yours may take longer. Watch closely and do the snap test on* **each piece** *of placenta. The umbilical cord keepsake may take an additional 1-2 hours to dehydrate. Food dehydrators vary greatly in dehydration times. Follow your manufacturer's recommendations if you choose to use a food dehydrator instead of your oven.*

6
PART 6: BEGINNING PHASE 2 OF THE ENCAPSULATION PROCESS!

(Allow 1-3 hours to grind and encapsulate the placenta, depending on if you choose to grind by hand or use an electric grinder.)

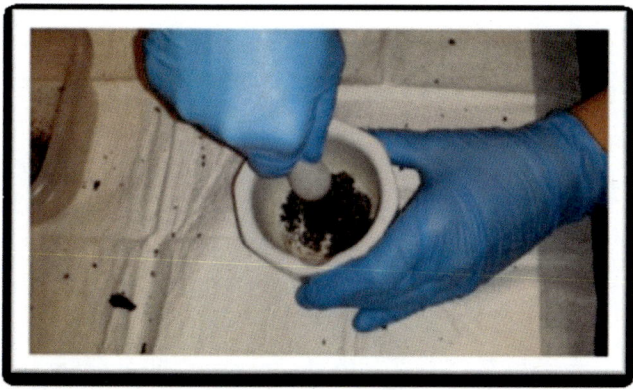

Step 43: Place a small amount of placenta into the mortar and pestle, roughly 1 tbsp. (alternatively, you could use an electric grinder for faster grinding if you prefer.)

Begin by pressing gently directly down on the placenta pieces. Increase force gradually, so as not to cause the placenta to jump out of the mortar. Once the larger pieces are broken up, begin grinding against the edges of the bowl in a circular motion. You are done with a batch of grinding when the granules are roughly the size of sea salt.

A small amount of placenta is much easier to pound and grind!
Doing several small batches of grinding is much faster and less frustrating than placing a large amount of placenta in the mortar and pestle. You may wish to watch Powerful Mamas YouTube video on using a mortar and pestle effectively for grinding placenta, found on www.PowerfulMamas.com/blog.

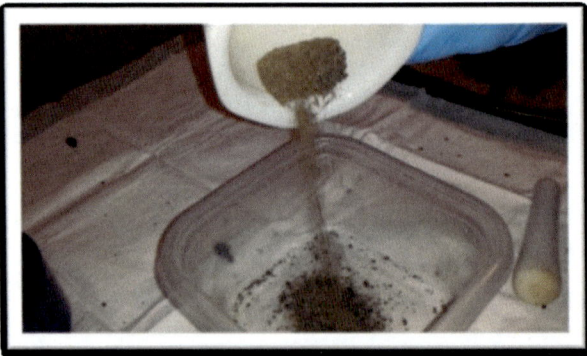

Step 44: Continue Grinding in Small Batches, Placing the Finished Powder into a Small Bowl. Continue until all of the Placenta is Pulverized and Ready to be Placed into Capsules.

KEEP IN MIND YOU MAY CHOOSE TO SKIP ENCAPSULATION AND ADD THE GROUND PLACENTA POWDER DIRECTLY TO FOOD OR SMOOTHIES!

Step 45: While Grinding You May Notice Hard, White Pieces. These Are Likely Calcium Deposits.

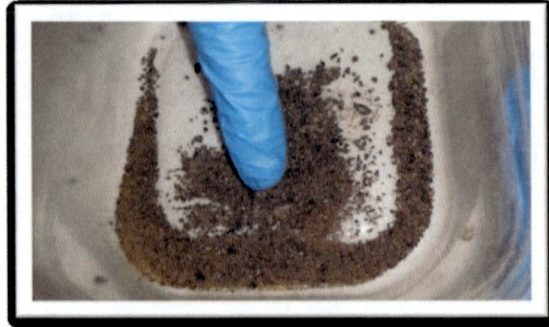

You can encapsulate small calcium deposits, but larger pieces should be thrown away. (Calcium deposits are more numerous on gestationally-older placentas.)

Step 46: Locate Empty Capsules.

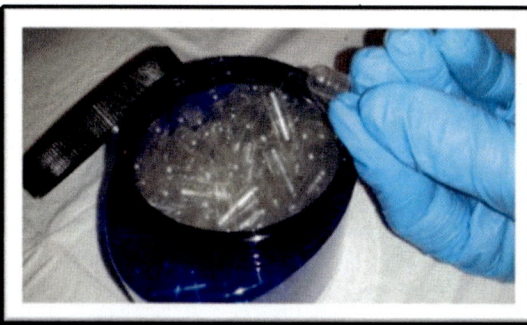

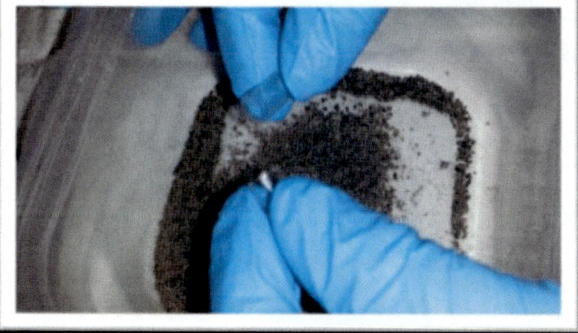

Step 47: Open Each Capsule. If Filling by Hand, Scoop Each Side of the Capsule into the Placenta Powder. Firmly Close Each Capsule by Placing the Long and Short End Together.

*If Using an Encapsulation Machine, Follow the Manufacturer's Provided Directions.

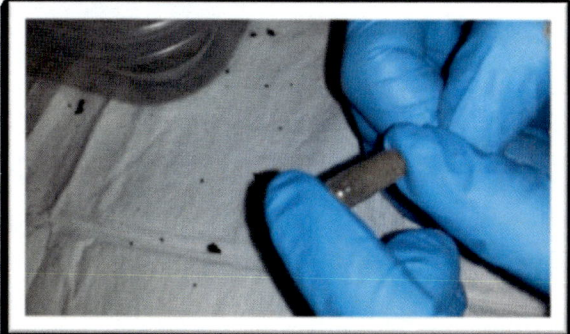

Place finished capsules into a dark jar. You may wish to mark the jar with the quantity of capsules the placenta yielded and the date the encapsulation was completed. **Consider adding a food safe desiccant packet to the jar to reduce humidity. If you need to pause during the encapsulation process, place the grinded placenta powder in a bowl with a lid in a cool, dark location. You may come back to it later to finish.**

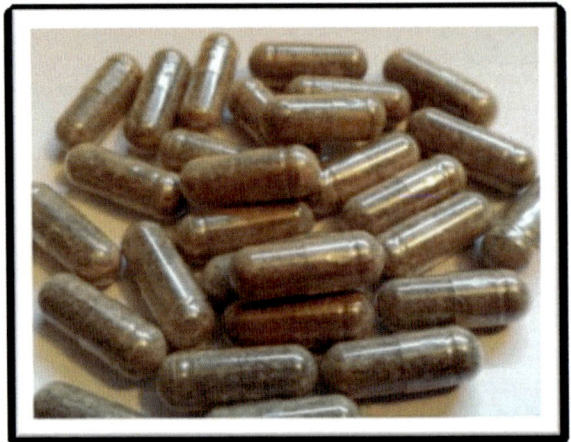

Step 48: Enjoy the Fruits of Your Labor!!! ☺ Follow the advice of your medical provider and listen to how your body is feeling regarding dosage. A suggested daily intake might be 1-2 capsules, 2-3 times daily the first 2-3 weeks postpartum, decreasing consumption until all capsules are gone. Raw preparations of the placenta are generally more potent than basic-heated capsules. Hormones begin to break down after 6-12 months, so you may want to use all of your capsules by that point. Many women choose to save their placenta tincture for long-term use.

***Ground placenta can be stored in a cool, dark place up to 6 weeks, but then any remaining powder or capsules should be moved into a freezer. Alternatively, they could be placed directly into the freezer. Capsules should NOT be kept in the fridge – the humidity levels can lead to spoilage!!!

POWERFUL MAMAS HEALING PLACENTA SALVE RECIPE

Ingredients:

2 TB. Shea Butter

1 TB. Coconut Oil

1 Tsp. Calendula Oil or 1 TB Calendula Dried Leaves

1 Tsp. Plantain Leaf Extract or 1 TB Dried Leaves

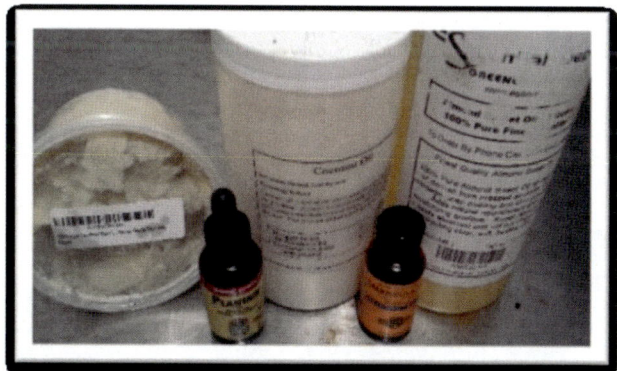

5 Drops Therapeutic Grade Lavender Essential Oil

2 Drops Therapeutic Grade Tea Tree Essential Oil

1 TB. Beeswax – (Optional, adds firmness)

1 TB. Ground Placenta Powder

Directions: Place all ingredients in a small crockpot on low heat for 2 hours. Strain salve through a coffee filter to remove granules. Pour into a container with a reliable seal. You may keep your salve in the refrigerator or freezer for a firmer consistency.

POWERFUL MAMAS PLACENTA SMOOTHIE RECIPE

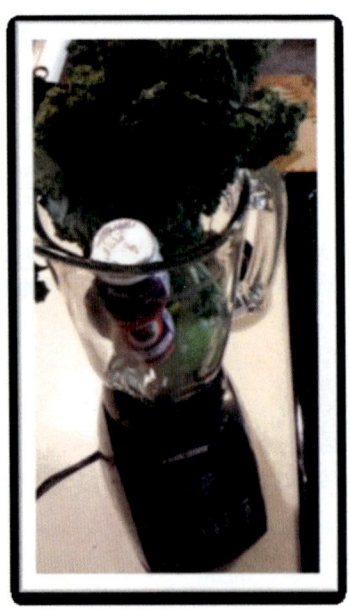

Ingredients:

2 Ice Cube-Sized Chunks of Rinsed, FRESH, Raw Placenta from the Maternal Side Only OR 1 TB. Dried Placenta Powder

1 Cup Ice Cubes

1 Cup Almond Milk

1 Cup Greek Yogurt

1 Banana

½ Cup Strawberries

1 Cup Chopped Kale

Directions: Place all ingredients in blender & pulverize. Feel free to alter this recipe to fit your own preferences. If using fresh placenta, make sure it is no more than 24 hours old, or has been frozen within 24 hours of the birth.

ABOUT THE AUTHOR

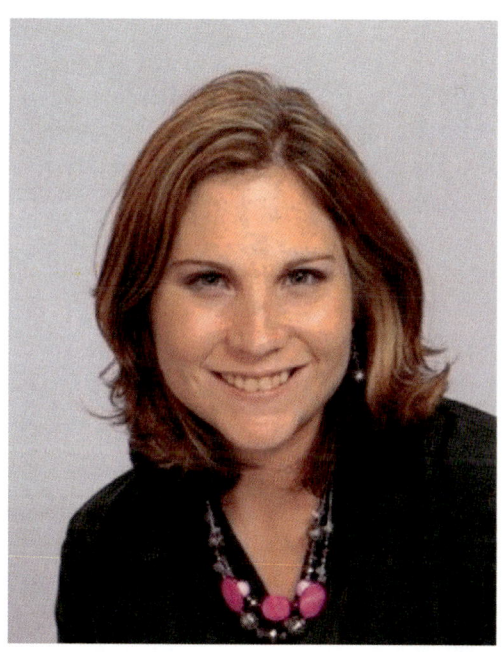

Jacquelyn Duke, owner of Powerful Mamas®, believes EVERY woman has incredible, undeniable strength. With the right support, education, and perhaps a few innovative products, mamas can have an empowering pregnancy, birth, and postpartum experience!

Aside from being a mother, (her most important career), Jacquelyn's passion is helping others understand their choices and find their own inner power during childbirth. Jacquelyn has been teaching natural childbirth education classes both online and to a full and boisterous room since 2011 through Powerful Mamas®. She has had the distinct honor of supporting families as a labor doula since 2010. She enjoys being able to use her advocacy experience from her former careers on Capitol Hill and as a Paralegal as she comes alongside families during their pregnancies and labor experiences. Her Master's Degree in Education comes in handy, along with her CAPPA CCCE and CLD certifications when she is educating families on their birthing options. However, she is quick to tell you that the most valuable education she has received by far is from the amazing women she has been blessed to work with over the years. Each of their births has taught her something new and powerful!

Jacquelyn is married to a wonderful man who is a loving husband and a great daddy! With the guidance of a doula, he supported her through her own natural, drug-free childbirths; one at the hospital and one a lovely water birth at home. Their two little girls are the light of their world!

DISCLAIMER

This content is not intended to be a substitute for professional medical advice, diagnosis, or treatment. Always seek the advice of your physician or other qualified health provider with any questions you may have regarding a medical condition. Never disregard professional medical advice or delay in seeking it. **Follow the recommendation of your physician or other qualified health provider regarding the safety of consuming your placenta. Conditions at the time of birth and storage procedures can affect the safety of consuming the placenta!** Never allow anyone other than the mother that produced the placenta to consume the placenta. Powerful Mamas highly recommends that the mother prepare the placenta herself, to avoid spreading illness or disease via blood borne pathogens.

Reliance on any information provided by Powerful Mamas or Intrinsic Birthing LLC is solely at your own risk. Buyer assumes all risk and responsibility associated with preparing and consuming the placenta. Any statements or claims about the possible health benefits conferred by Placenta Encapsulation, Placenta Pills, Placenta Tinctures, Placenta Balms, or any other foods or supplements for which instructional guides are sold by Powerful Mamas or Intrinsic Birthing LLC have not been evaluated by the Food & Drug Administration and are not intended to diagnose, treat, cure or prevent any disease.

Copyright 2014 Intrinsic Birthing LLC, All Rights Reserved

Made in the USA
Las Vegas, NV
11 August 2023